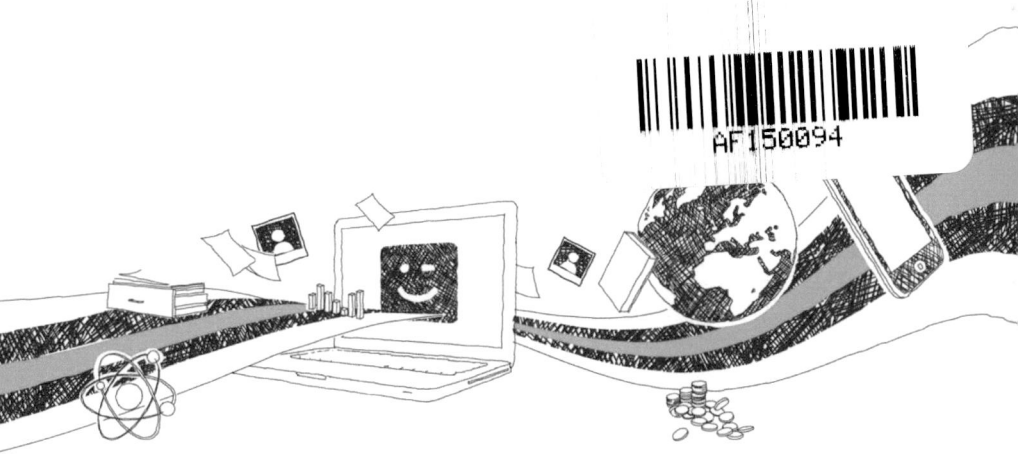
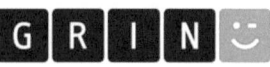

Carol Benjamin

Types of Designs in Health Research

GRIN Publishing

Bibliographic information published by the German National Library:

The German National Library lists this publication in the National Bibliography; detailed bibliographic data are available on the Internet at http://dnb.dnb.de .

Imprint:

Copyright © 2011 GRIN Verlag GmbH
Print and binding: Books on Demand GmbH, Norderstedt Germany
ISBN: 978-3-656-55451-6

This book at GRIN:

http://www.grin.com/en/e-book/265789/types-of-designs-in-health-research

GRIN - Your knowledge has value

Since its foundation in 1998, GRIN has specialized in publishing academic texts by students, college teachers and other academics as e-book and printed book. The website www.grin.com is an ideal platform for presenting term papers, final papers, scientific essays, dissertations and specialist books.

Visit us on the internet:

http://www.grin.com/

http://www.facebook.com/grincom

http://www.twitter.com/grin_com

Types of Designs in Health Research

By

Carol Benjamin

Trident University

Abstract

This assignment describes the two types of analytic study types in health research. Observational study which includes cross sectional, case-control and cohort are discussed. Randomized controlled trials are briefly discussed as an example of experimental study design. The three major research designs are describes, contrasted and discussed as well as the strengths and limitations.

Types of Designs in Health Research

In conducting a research study in health research or other areas of interest, it is very important to choose the correct design since the method chosen could affect the results and also the findings. Research approach follows research problems: the appropriate research approach is the one that best fits with your research problem (Bloomberg & Volpe (2008). The goal of all researchers is to have reliable observation which will give a better understanding of the problem to be studied.

In health research, there are various types of design that are available for researcher to conduct their studies. Once the researcher identifies the research question the next step will be the selection of a research design. There are two broad areas of analytic study types in health research and they are described as experimental and observational methods.

Randomized controlled trials are associated with experimental design in health research. Stolberg, Norman & Trop (2004) state that randomized controlled trial is one of the simplest but most powerful tools of research. In essence, the randomized controlled trial is a study in which people are allocated at random to receive one of several clinical interventions. The authors also state that "intervention" refers to treatment, but it should be used in a much wider sense to include any clinical maneuver offered to study participants that may have an effect on their health status. Such clinical maneuvers include prevention strategies, screening programs, diagnostic tests, interventional procedures, the setting in which health care is provided, and educational models.

Stolberg, Norman & Trop (2004) explain that randomized controlled trials are used to examine the effect of interventions on particular outcomes such as death or the

3

recurrence of disease. The authors state that some consider randomized controlled trials to be the best of all research designs, or "the most powerful tool in modern clinical research", mainly because the act of randomizing patients to receive or not receive the intervention ensures that, on average, all other possible causes are equal between the two groups.

Shlipak & Stehman-Breen (2005) argue that observational, patient oriented research is a broad term used to describe clinical studies that do not involve an experiment or intervention, in contrast to clinical trials. The traditional study designs of epidemiology case series, cross-sectional analysis, case-control, and cohort studies are all examples of observational research. The authors also argue that this type of research can be designed and implemented by a primary data collection, meaning that the investigator recruits the subjects and conducts the measurement by him or her. However the authors state that data collection is an expensive and lengthy process that limits the feasibility of addressing many research questions and would hinder many potential investigators from engaging in research.

The three observational analytic research types are discussed in more detail in this assignment. These studies are referred to as "observational" since the researcher simply observes and no interventions are carried out by the investigator (Mann, 2003).

Cohort Studies

These are the best method for determining the incidence and natural history of a condition. The studies may be prospective or retrospective and some times two cohorts are compare (Mann, 2003). The author explains that in prospective cohort studies, a group of people is chosen who do not have the outcome of interest (for example,

4

myocardial infraction). Over a period of time the people in the sample are observed to see whether they develop the outcome of interest (that is, myocardial infarction).

Mann explained that in single cohort studies, those people who do not develop the outcome of interest are used as internal controls. Mann (2003) also describes retrospective cohort studies and explains that this method use data already collected for other purposes. The methodology is the same as in prospective cohort studies, and the cohort is "followed up retrospectively". The study period may be many years but the time to complete the study is only as long as it takes to collect and analyze the data.

Mann (2003) explains many advantages (strengths) and disadvantages (limitations) of cohort studies. He states that a single study can examine various outcome variables. For example, cohort studies can simultaneously look at death from lung, cardiovascular, and cerebrovascular disease. The author made a contrast with case-control studies as they assess only one outcome variable. That is, the outcome initially entered in the case.

Mann also argues that retrospective studies are much cheaper as the data have already been collected. One advantage of such a study design is the lack of bias because the current interest was not the original reason for the data to be collected. However, because the cohort was originally constructed for another purpose it is unlikely that all the relevant information will have been rigorously collected. Mann also explained that retrospective cohorts also suffer the disadvantage that people with the outcome of interest are more likely to remember certain antecedents, or exaggerate or minimize what they now consider to be risk factors (recall bias).

Cross-Sectional Studies

Mann (2003) explains that cross-sectional studies are primarily used to determine prevalence which equals the number of cases in a population at a given point in time. All the measurements on each person are made at one point in time. Article written by Blast (2011) states that cross-sectional studies gather information about the prevalence of health-related states and conditions. All they can do is measure the frequency (prevalence) of conditions and demonstrate associations. They cannot identify cause-and-effect relationships, though they do identify the existence of health problems.

Blast also states that cross-sectional studies, also known as surveys, are a useful way to gather information on important health-related aspects of people's knowledge, attitudes, and practices. The author also shows the distinction between a cohort study and a repeated cross-sectional study. He states that a cohort study is conducted with the same individuals who participate over a long period, repeated or serial cross-sectional studies do not study the same individuals repeatedly.

Mann (2003) explains the advantages (strengths) and disadvantages (limitations) of cross sectional studies and states that this method is quick and cheap. Since there are no follow-up, less resources are required to run the study. This method is the best way to determine prevalence and is useful at identifying associations that can then be more rigorously studied using a cohort study. Mann also states that the most important problem with cross sectional studies is differentiating cause and effect or the sequence of events. Rare conditions cannot efficiently be studied using cross sectional studies because even in large samples there may be no one with the disease. So in this situation it is better to study a cross sectional sample of patients who already have the disease.

Case-Control Studies

In contrast with cohort and cross-sectional studies, case control studies are usually retrospective. People with the outcome of interest are matched with a control group who do not. Retrospectively the researcher determines which individuals were exposed to the agent or treatment or the prevalence of a variable in each of the study groups. Where the outcome is rare, case- control studies may be the only feasible approach (Mann, 2003).

Mann (2003) explains that since some of the subjects have been deliberately chosen because they have the disease in question, case-control studies are much more cost effective than cohort and cross sectional studies. Mann also argued that case-control studies determine the relative importance of a predictor variable in relation to the presence or absence of the disease. Case-control studies are retrospective and cannot be used to calculate the relative risk. This is a prospective cohort study. Case-control studies can however be used to calculate odds ratio, which in turn, usually approximate to the relative risk.

Mann explains the advantages (strengths) and disadvantages (limitations) of case-control studies. He states that when condition is uncommon, case-control studies generate a lot of information from relatively few subjects. When there is a long latent period between an exposure and the disease, case-control studies are the only feasible option. In case-control study comparatively few subjects are required so more resources are available for studying each. In consequence a huge number of variables can be considered. This type of study is therefore useful for generating hypotheses that can be tested using other types of study.

The major problems with case-controls study are confounding variables and bias. Bias may take two major forms:

1. Sampling - the patient with the disease may be a biased sample. (for example, patients referred to a teaching hospital) or the control may be biased (for example, volunteers, different ages, sex or socioeconomic group).

2. Observation and recall bias - As the study assesses predictor variables retrospectively there is a great potential for a biased assessment of their presence and significance by the patient or the investigator, or both (Mann, 2003).

References

Bloomberg, L., Volpe, M. (2008). Completing your Qualitative Dissertation. A
Roadmap from Beginning to End. Thousand Oaks, CA: Sage.

Last, J. (2011). Cross Sectional Study. Retrieved on April 29, 2011 from:
http://www.enotes.com/public-health-encyclopedia/cross-sectional-study

Mann, C. J. (2003). Observational research methods. Research design II: cohort, cross
sectional, and case-control studies. Emergency Medicine Journal. 20: 54-60.

Shlipak, M., Stehman-Breen, C. (2005). Observational Research Databases in Renal
disease. Retrieved on April 29, 2011 from:
http://jasn.asnjournals.org/content/16/12/3477.full.pdf

Stolberg, H., Norman, G., Trop, I. (2004). Fundamentals of Clinical Research for
Radiologists. Randomized Controlled Trials. American Journal of Roentgenology.
183: 1539-1544.